NATURAL COMPLETE GUIDE TO ACNE ERADICATION

Easiest Way Of Healing Acne

PETER MORRISON

All Rights Reserved:

Without the publisher's prior written consent, no part of this publication may be copied, distributed, or transmitted in any way, including by photocopying, recording, or other electronic or mechanical methods, except for brief quotations used in critical reviews and other noncommercial uses allowed by copyright law.

Copyrights © (PETER MORRISON), 2022

DISCLAIMER

The author of this book collaborates with medical professionals but is not a doctor or a nurse. Any advice in this book should not be implemented without first consulting a medical expert. This book's information is not meant to be a replacement for qualified medical guidance, diagnosis, or care. Always ask your doctor or dermatologist for help if you have any concerns about a medical problem.

TABLE OF CONTENT

INTRODUCTION

You've already tried all of those cures, quick fixes, treatments, and lotions, which is the problem. Spending a small sum on acne treatments has put you through the wringer, and now you're perplexed and angry that you aren't seeing the same results that everyone else does.

I'm delighted to let you know that your continuous acne suffering is going to come to an end, forever, as someone who had endured severe acne for a long time.

I eventually conquered my acne beast after years of trial and error, testing, spending thousands of dollars on therapies, and working with cutting-edge medical professionals and skilled dermatologists.

While it took me several years to realise that the vast majority of treatments and products that are aggressively pushed on those of us who suffer from acne can exacerbate our acne and lead to excessive breakouts, it took me even longer to reach the point in my life when acne was history. Grab a drink, turn off the television, and prepare for an eye-opening exploration of the myriad approaches available for taking back control of your life and permanently curing acne.

Have a good time reading!

WHAT IS ACNE?

(Acne: The Real Story)

Skin follicles become clogged with oil and dead skin cells, resulting in a skin disorder known as acne.

Most people have dealt with acne at some point in their lives, particularly during adolescence when sebaceous glands are producing more oil than usual. Adult acne, on the other hand, has no age restrictions, and it affects a lot of people in their 40s and 50s.

There are a lot of myths regarding what causes acne and why some individuals get it while others don't, living acne-free lives without ever having to feel the discomfort of severe acne.

An additional set of issues are brought on by these myths and absurd ideas. People with acne are so desperate to get rid of it that they try all kinds of unconventional methods, such as changing their diet or over-tanning in the hope that it will permanently reduce pimples.

When used improperly, these treatments can undermine your efforts to manage your acne and, in many instances, may even exacerbate your condition. These "quick cure cures" can have the unintended consequence of leaving lifelong scars.

What exactly is acne, then?

To begin with, despite what you may have heard, acne is not fatal, and no one has ever died. According to clinical terminology, a hormonal imbalance—which is sometimes referred to as "chronic inflammation" or "systemic inflammation" in medicine—causes acne.Poor digestion, combined with an unhealthy diet, is the leading cause of chronic inflammation.

Your body's pores getting clogged, typically on your face, neck, upper body, back, and even chest is another major factor in acne development.

The intensity and extent of the skin damage brought on by the various varieties of acne fall into five distinct categories:

Comedones
Papule
Pustule
Nodule
Cyst

Cysts are categorised as belonging to the nodule category while comedones, which include blackheads and whiteheads, are regarded as being acne symptoms.

"Acne Vulgaris" is another name for acne, a type of it that typically develops during adolescence.

The back, face, and chest are its main target areas. Among teenage boys and girls, acne vulgaris is a problem. Between the ages of 17 and 20, over 50–70% of teenage guys are impacted. Between the ages of 15 and 18, girls are typically affected.

The severity of your acne can be estimated by looking at how different groups of people describe acne:

Heads of Black
If your pores are partially clogged and some of the bacteria, dead skin cells and sebum can escape and drain to the surface of your skin, you will get blackheads.

Consistently cleaning your face will not stop blackheads from developing because the dark colour that goes along with them is not dirt. Blackheads are more solid and frequently take a few days to a week to disappear.

Whitish Heads

Whiteheads, the reverse of a black head, will show up when a pore is entirely plugged.

Whiteheads are a temporary condition brought on by trapped sebum, germs, and dead skin cells beneath the skin's surface.

Papules

These pimples are throbbingly painful, red, inflamed, and headless.Pustules What we often refer to as "pimples" are pustules. Despite always being inflamed and having a white or yellow centre, they resemble white heads quite a bit.

Nodules Because of how painful they may be, nodules, which are bigger spots, might remain for months. Under the skin's surface, nodules are hardened lumps, and scarring is frequently associated with nodules.

If you think you have nodules, please do not squeeze them as doing so may severely harm your skin, cause the nodules to spread, and prolong your life.

Nodules are very challenging to manage with over-the-counter medications or homemade cures, so don't attempt to treat them yourself. Instead, schedule a consultation with your dermatologist for advice.

Cysts
Cysts can be big and feel hard, just like nodules can. Some cysts can feel like round balls under the skin.

In addition, they are liquid-filled and quite painful. The bacteria and infection may spread deeper into your skin if you crush or attempt to rupture a cyst.In addition to the four types of acne that are regarded to be more severe and require medical attention, there are also the typical forms of acne that many of us have seen occasionally during our lives.

Globular acne
The emergence of multiple big nodules, many of which are joined and interconnected and include a significant number of blackheads, characterises this severe form of acne. These lesions have the potential

to turn into ulcers, which results in severely scarred skin that is disfiguring.

The face, back, chest, upper arms, and thighs are the typical locations for conglobata.

Acne conglobata is more prevalent in men and typically affects people between the ages of 18 and 30.

It should be mentioned that Acne Conglobata can persist for many years before going dormant and reappearing when a certain event takes place. Acne Conglobata's origin is still uncertain.

Ulcerative acne
This kind of severe acne truly manifests suddenly and typically affects young guys.

The severe nodulocystic acne symptoms, which frequently include ulceration, are obvious. The lesions are widespread on the extremities and the facial region, just like in typical cases of acne, and may eventually leave behind unsightly scars.

However, acne is distinct since it also includes fever-like symptoms, hurting joints, especially in the knees and hips, and variable amounts of weight loss that vary from person to person.

Gram-negative folliculitis
A severe form of acne called gram-negative folliculitis is brought on by bacterial infection-induced follicular inflammation:

Cysts and pustules are the primary symptoms of this illness.

In certain instances, it has been found that the development of the condition is brought on by a side effect of treating acne vulgaris with antibiotics for a prolonged period.

Gram is a type of blue stain used in scientific tests for microscopic organisms, which is why this type of acne is known as "gram-negative." The term "gram-negative" refers to bacteria that do not stain blue.

Gram-negative folliculitis is an uncommon condition that, like other forms of severe or intense acne, affects both sexes equally, thus we are unsure of whether it affects men or women more frequently.

Face Pyoderma

Only females experience this sort of severe acne, and they typically range in age from 20 to 40.

Large, painful nodules, pustules, and sores with the potential for scarring are its defining features.

Pyoderma can develop suddenly and affect a woman's skin even if she's never had acne before.

The majority of the time, this severe acne just affects the face, and although it seldom lasts longer than a year, it may still do a lot of harm in a short amount of time.

Although it can affect both sexes, men are more likely than women to develop the acne-like condition known as keloidalis.The neck area is frequently impacted by keloidalis. The skin becomes extremely oily and develops atrophic scars and keloids on the neck, shoulders, and upper back as the inflamed papules and pustules develop into larger cysts and nodules.

Acne of other sorts includes:

*Acne Rosacea: This condition, which is most prevalent in older people, is characterised by red rashes on the chin, nose, cheeks, and forehead.

*Acne Conglobata: This severe inflammatory condition features comedones, nodules, abscesses, and sinus drainage tracts.

*Acne fulminans is a severe form of the skin condition acne that can develop following a failed attempt to treat another kind of acne, such as acne. However, adults are not immune to acne, and those of us who do not treat it can wind up having it for the rest of our lives. Acne typically affects people during their adolescent years.

EXAMINING THE ROOT CAUSES OF ACNE

Acne appears when oil and dead skin cells clog the pores on your skin.

A sebaceous gland, which produces the greasy substance known as sebum, is connected to each pore. P. acnes, also known as Propionibacterium acnes, can grow more quickly when sebum buildup plugs pores.

Whiteheads, blackheads, and pimples are typical symptoms of acne, while some cases are more severe than others.

Numerous factors can affect acne formation, including:

genetics

diet

stress

hormonal changes

infections.

However, several influencing factors, such as the following, are regularly associated to both acne sufferers and those without it.

Puberty

Even those of us who have never had acne before (or afterwards) have experienced the telltale signs and symptoms of breakouts at this time, which is when teenagers and pimples always seem to go hand in hand.

Over 94% of people between the ages of 12 and 24 have suffered acne at some point in their life, according to studies.

Teenage acne is so common because of the hormone androgens, which begin to function excessively as we get closer to puberty.

Our skin pores and hair follicles may become more oily as a result of androgens. The oil can clog our pores and cause temporary acne outbreaks when it interacts with the skin cells on our bodies.

Their Hormones

Hormones have consistently been linked to the emergence of severe acne in both teenagers and adults, suggesting that they may play a critical role in the development of acne.

Family Comes First

Despite the fact that acne is not directly inherited, it has been said that the likelihood of you developing acne is greatly increased if one of your parents suffered from severe acne. There is currently no concrete evidence of a causal connection between parents and children who have acne, but researchers are still looking into the topic.

Your Prescriptions

Certain prescription pharmaceuticals, particularly antidepressants and anxiety medications, as well as specific types of steroids, barbiturates, and lithium, have been known to aggravate acne depending on the medication you are taking.

If you are taking any drugs and believe they are making your acne worse, talk to your doctor about any prescription-only options you can use to prevent this.

DO NOT discontinue taking your medication prior to speaking with your healthcare provider.

Our Surroundings

If you've been exposed to chemicals at work or even at home with household cleaners, air fresheners, or scented detergents, your pre-existing acne can become momentarily worse.

There have also been case studies where people who had never had acne began breaking out severely after being exposed to chemical cleaners on a regular basis, especially when cleaning without gloves.

ALTERNATIVE (NATURAL) TREATMENT FOR ACNE

Natural, holistic, or at-home acne treatment solutions can be reasonably priced.

Natural and herbal remedies are made from thriving plants. You may have noticed that a vitamin supplement tastes like leaves, ground plants, or anything similar just before swallowing if you've ever taken one. There are no chemicals used.

Natural herbal remedies don't trick your body, mess with the chemical makeup of the brain, or mess with the hormone balance.

Why? Because the herbs possess certain properties that are meant to regulate biological functions and promote healing and good health.

They are neither artificial or man-made; they simply sprung from the earth and are present to assist with the problems we face. It is beneficial to take natural supplements rather than prescription drugs.

A list of many natural treatments is provided below.

*Drinks high in antioxidants, vitamin C, and/or vitamin E can help repair and revive the skin.

Vitamin E-rich foods can lessen acne scars.

A common DIY treatment for acne is tea tree oil. It is a diluted essential oil that is used topically to treat acne blemishes. Tea tree oil has the ability to destroy germs, therefore applying it topically to acne lesions is thought to eliminate the acne-causing bacteria.

Additionally, some herbs that may be ingested help treat chronic inflammatory issues, particularly those that affect the skin, like acne.

These herbs include the blue flag, echinacea, cleavers, red clover, figwort, burdock, and cleavers. The herbs blue flag, burdock, yellow dock, and echinacea go well together. Tea can be made by combining these and infusing them with hot water.

3 times a day, consume a cup of this. To improve the flavour, add a little honey to it.

Always concentrate on drugs or ointments that include Benzoyl peroxide 5 percent while researching over-the-counter options.

Before going to bed every day, apply this to your trouble areas.

Benzoyl helps with open sores and pimples, as well as unclogging blackheads and getting rid of the germs that frequently live in your skin's pores. Just a fingertip's worth should be plenty for your needs.

When used on the skin, benzoyl peroxide effectively destroys bacteria, dries the skin, and encourages the production of new cells.

Lower doses are available over the counter, but prescription medication is needed for stronger levels.

Here are a couple of my go-to natural treatments for acne that works quickly:

Compresses, Both Hot And Cold

This is a straightforward home remedy that is among the most well-liked. To treat acne on your face, chest, or back, all you have to do is moisten a cloth and rub it against the affected region.

This will lessen swelling and immediately clear blocked pores, which is a major factor in the development of acne.

Organic Fruit Juice

Utilising natural fruit juices as a means of reducing the presence of external cysts and uncomfortable blackheads is one straightforward yet efficient technique.

By combining some cucumber or citrus fruit juice with some almond oil, you can apply these juices topically.

Apply the mixture to the entire acne-affected region and let it sit for 15 minutes. Rinse with warm water, then pat yourself dry.

Regular application of almond oil and similar natural ingredients is an effective home remedy for clearing up acne.

As long as they are natural and free of added sugars or sweeteners, you can also use lemon or apricot juice in place of cucumber juice.

Treatment with Fenugreek Leaf

Fenugreek leaves help keep acne from coming back once you have it under control rather than treating acne. To make a paste, simply add water to a small bowl with the crushed leaves.

Use this as a face mask and keep it on for the entire night. Use an old pillowcase to avoid light stains, as new ones can leave them.

The Honey Mask

Because of its inherent antibacterial properties, honey is frequently applied as a facemask in spas and at home. You may buy these masks at your neighbourhood drugstore for a reasonable price.

Enjoy the effects by using the mask once or twice a week. It functions incredibly well!

Treatment with White Vinegar

This is yet another topical remedy that is quite effective. White vinegar should be applied to the diseased area using a cotton ball after being soaked in it for 5 to 15 minutes.

Use cold water to wash off. Apply vinegar after diluting it with a third cup of water if you find it to be too powerful.

Mask with oats

Cook some plain oatmeal in little amounts, then spread it over your face. 15 minutes after applying this combination to your skin, rinse it off.

A natural exfoliant, oatmeal offers immediate comfort. As it requires little time and effort and produces excellent results, try to incorporate this strategy at least twice every week.

Yeast (Alternative) Solution

Apply to face, wait till it becomes hard (try not to move), peel off, or wash with warm water. Combine 1 tablespoon of dry or fresh yeast with 2 teaspoons of lemon juice.

Remedy with Bay Leaf

Apply bay leaves to your face after grinding them and blanching them in warm water. Ten minutes later, rinse.

Green (Alternative) Solution

Place clean, rinsed lettuce leaves in a bowl of water. Rinse the water off your face.

The Tea Bag Treatment

When the water is boiling, add some basil and two to three tea bags. With a clean cotton ball, apply the solution to the acne.

The natural treatments mentioned above have all been successfully employed throughout time.

I have discovered the honey mask to be effective, and the oatmeal mask mixture has helped me keep my acne under control without the need for pricey outside treatments.

HOW TO TREAT ACNE

There is no one-size-fits-all acne treatment due to the vast differences between different types of skin (oily, normal, dry, or combo skin).

For patients with acne who are above 12 years old, the FDA recently approved the use of a gel called Epiduo.

Epiduo, a mixture of two tried-and-true therapies for acne, is prescribed for single use daily. Epiduo contains the generic drug Differin, which is marketed as having Benzoyl peroxide 2.5% and Adapalene 0.1%.

The Epiduo gel, which for the first time combines the two, was announced by the product's makers, Galderma, in a recent press release. The gel is expected to be available in early 2009.

A vital element that fights acne is salicylic acid, which is found in several different over-the-counter drugs like Sri-dex, Clearasil, Clearstick, and Oxy Night Watch.

An effective retinoid called isotretinoin can be taken orally if the acne is extremely bad and a cyst has developed, rendering other drugs immune.

Additionally, it has become usual practice to prevent acne outbreaks by taking oral antibiotics. Initially strong doses of the antibiotics, which are then gradually reduced, aid in reducing the inflammation.

However, if the acne over time develops a resistance to the antibiotic, treatment will fail.

Acne has long been treated in the US with a variety of broad-spectrum antibiotics.

The best approach to figuring out what will work for you as a treatment is to see a dermatologist for a thorough evaluation.

Depending on the severity of your acne as well as your unique skin type, your dermatologist will be able to decide which treatment is ideal for you. Unbelievable (yet efficient) home remedies

Here are a few of my personal favourite natural acne treatments if you're ready to venture out and risk the odd, curious looks of friends and family who could catch you in the act.

IMPORTANT: All of these treatments are completely secure.

Solution Using Toothpaste

To be completely honest, I didn't think this home remedy would work when I initially read about it. I chose to give it a try anyhow because I had nothing to lose, and I'm pleased I did.

It not only takes just a few seconds to complete, but it also performs very effectively.

A small amount of your preferred toothpaste will do.

Your zits, sores, and acne spots should all receive a small amount, which you should leave on overnight to dry. Use an old pillowcase, please.

Baking soda and water can be used as a substitute for toothpaste.

All you need to do is rinse it off in the morning. When you have a painful breakout, do this two or three times per week.

The Aspirin Mask

Aspirin has been approved by dermatologists for use in the creation of a facemask that can help treat acne. This approach is risk-free and efficient, and it not only has the power to clear up acne but also lessen scarring that already exists!

To make your aspirin mask, follow these steps:

Elements:

    ☐ Honey

    ☐ Non coated aspirin (any brand)

    ☐ Neutrogena Healthy Skin Anti Wrinkle Cream

    ☐ Alcohol Free Skin Toner

Recipe:

1) Take four aspirin tablets and put them in a little bowl.

2) Drench the aspirin in water. Only add a few drops of water to loosen it; do not use more than that or the aspirin will disintegrate. Rub the aspirin and water together with your fingertips to thoroughly mix the two ingredients and separate the aspirin tablets.It should have a very gritty texture.

3) Lastly, stir in two teaspoons of honey to the mixture. Aspirin, water, and honey must all be well included in the mixture.

4) Do not let any of the mixtures get in your eyes while applying them to your face. Leave the aspirin mask on your face for 10 minutes after you've covered it completely.

Whenever something is on your face, avoid touching or rubbing it in. When the ten minutes are over, wash the mixture off your face with lukewarm water to remove the aspirin granules that were on your face while it was still wet (exfoliating your skin).

5) Use the toner to blot your face and smooth it all over once you've washed the oil from your skin. Additionally, by doing this, you'll get rid of any leftover formula, giving your face a fresh appearance.

6) As a finishing touch, polish your face with the moisturiser you bought and replenish the hydration. Retinol, which tightens your skin and lessens wrinkles and creases, should be in your moisturiser

3 or more times per week.

The Use Of Ice

Another simple at-home treatment that has always been effective when I've used it for severe outbreaks. Applying a cold compact (or a bag of broken ice) to your face each night before bed is all that is required.

A damp towel will also be effective because it will lessen swelling and aid in clearing up clogged pores that lead to breakouts.

Magnesium Milk (Three-Part Process)

This is a fantastic, completely safe cleaner that can be used at home. Apply it directly to the diseased region, then let it sit there for 10 to 15 minutes before rinsing.

Next, combine 3/4 cup of hot water with 1 teaspoon of Epsom salt (magnesium sulphate).

Apply with a clean towel to the affected area (avoid cotton balls as they may stick to the skin and cause blocked pores). After 20 minutes of application, rinse with cold water.

The third and last step entails making a toner at home. You merely need to mix 3 drops of peroxide or benzoin oil into a cup of cold water.

Use this solution to wash your face, then rinse.

Give this antibacterial treatment a try; it works great!

Sandalwood Extract

One teaspoon of turmeric and sandalwood powder is all that is required for this treatment.

Combine this with a tiny bit of white milk (any kind). Apply it liberally to affected areas and leave it on for 15 to 25 minutes. After rinsing with warm water,towel off.

It may take a few sessions for this to start working, but the results are amazing. Again, you are free to repeat as often as you like.

THE OILED-UP APPROACH

This is one of the best techniques I've ever used, and I used to do it daily when my severe acne would flare up.

This acne-free formula only requires a little bottle of castor oil and a smaller bottle of extra virgin olive oil or, in a pinch, Jojoba oil. Your skin will receive moisture from virgin oil, which will help pull out any bacteria that may be hiding beneath the skin's surface.

Additionally, virgin oil will strengthen your skin with its built-in antioxidants.

Mix equal amounts of castor oil and olive oil to make a mixture. Starting with an equal blend of half and half is always advised, but you can experiment with different portions afterward.

Once everything is combined, carefully massage it over your body's afflicted areas (you can use this anywhere you like including your face, neck, upper body, and back). After applying it evenly to all of your diseased regions, cover it with a warm compress, like a towel or washcloth, and leave it there for 10 to 15 minutes.

This causes your face to naturally steam, which allows your pores to breathe and open up, eliminating toxins that are trapped beneath the skin's surface.

Leave the mixture on your body for ten to fifteen minutes while the compact acts as a sealer. After that, reapply the oils to your skin and rinse with cold water (not warm, as cold will tighten your skin and close your pores).

If you decide to use olive oil, be sure to get extra virgin rather than normal because it contains fewer contaminants. Jojoba oil is a great alternative to olive oil and can be used in its place as well.

A Vitamin A Day Prevents Acne
By ensuring that your skin receives appropriate nutrients and that your body is not creating excessive amounts of sebum, taking a multivitamin daily can help control acne (which is responsible for clogging pores).

A further helpful suggestion is to include chromium in your diet, a vitamin designed to treat skin problems.

TREATING (REMOVING) ACNE SCARS

There are steps you may take to decrease and remove scarring if acne has left you with an excessive amount of scarring.

One of these choices is a corrective surgical procedure called laser resurfacing, which is carried out in a hospital or medical facility by a doctor or dermatologist and will swiftly remove the look of scarring. Using this method, the top layer of your skin is removed to show a scar-free, spotless new layer beneath.

Similar to laser eye surgery, when a tiny layer of damaged tissue is removed to reveal a new, unharmed layer, any scarring or damage is immediately corrected and erased.

The associated fees are the only drawback to this technique. Resurfacing is a guaranteed way to completely remove scarring brought on by severe acne, but it can be highly expensive.

The punch graft treatment is used to treat severe acne scars. In this case, scarred skin is replaced with healthy, excellent skin that was taken from other regions of the body and grafted onto the area.
For a free consultation if you're curious to learn more about these procedures, get in touch with a dermatologist in your area.
The only surefire way to get rid of scarring that won't fade over time is with laser resurfacing, while there are also at-home methods that can help.
You can finish one of these treatments by applying Vitamin E to the scarred region. You can buy Vitamin E as a liquid or as a capsule from which you can cut the top to release the vitamin, which you can then apply to your scarred regions.
Additionally, virgin olive oil, which has been said to help lessen the look of scars, can be applied routinely to your scars.

TYPICAL ACNE MYTHS

Even though many of the old wives' stories concerning acne's causes have been debunked by experts, people nevertheless hold onto them. We'll try to dispel some of those persistent myths and put your mind at ease so you can continue on your path to clean, acne-free, flawless skin.

Myth: Acne only affects filthy individuals.
Factual statement: Hormonal changes occurring within the body, not inadequate cleanliness, are what cause acne. The sebaceous glands, which keep our skin moist, can occasionally overproduce oil to the point that they obstruct neighbouring hair follicles. As a result, the pores become clogged, leading to acne, which manifests as pimples, zits, pustules, and even cysts.

The truth is that routinely washing and scrubbing your skin can significantly exacerbate your acne condition. To properly care for your skin, you should wash it gently and pat it dry (not rubbing it).

Myth: People who have acne don't eat the right foods.
Experts now understand that there is no link between the meals you consume and the onset of acne.

The misconceptions that say chocolate and other fatty foods cause acne are false. However, if you want to have excellent overall health, you must practice good nutrition.

Myth: Acne results from stress
Acne can appear as a side effect of taking medications that are meant to help you deal with stress, but stress itself does not cause it. Consult your doctor to find out if the drug could be causing your skin problem if you use this kind of medication and experience acne symptoms like pimples, zits, or pustules. One word of warning: stress can exacerbate acne if you already have it even if it won't create it.

Myth: Acne is only a cosmetic issue.
Acne can affect your mental health in addition to changing how you look. Serious acne issues can result in severe acne and leave behind lifelong scars.

Severe acne is frequently characterised by cystic nodules and persistent outbreaks.

People's psychological well-being might occasionally be impacted by this when their self-image is altered. Many people experience issues with their self-worth and experience frustration and depression.

Myth: Acne cannot be cured.
Factual statement: By using the several products available and selecting the best therapy for your circumstances, acne can be cleared up.

Your dermatologist can identify the type of acne you have—whether it is acne vulgaris, cystic acne, nodular acne, or even rosacea—and help you choose the best course of treatment. Accutane, Retin-A, and many other medications are among the good, efficient therapies and pharmaceuticals that are accessible to assist resolve even the most enduring issues. You will soon unveil the stunning skin you were always destined to have.

MEDICATION FOR ACNE TREATMENT

Both topical and systemic medications are available to treat acne.

While systemic drugs are taken orally, topical treatments are applied to the skin. By treating the causes of acne's occurrence, the drugs' primary goal is to eradicate acne at its source.

The following medications are used to treat acne.

To treat acne, oral antibiotics are frequently used. The majority of the time, this is given to those who have persistent acne.

However, the acne-causing bacteria may quickly develop a resistance to the antibiotics and stop responding to treatment. The doctors will then typically recommend a new round of antibiotics to treat the problem. Erythromycin and tetracycline and their variants are the most often used antibiotic types.

However, erythromycin causes stomach pain, and tetracycline and its derivatives should not be used by expectant mothers or young children under the age of eight. These antibiotics' active ingredients treat the pustule or edema by internally drying it up.

Another class of drugs used to treat acne is topical retinoids. They are made from vitamin A and can stop the pores from closing. In reality, they prevent acne from forming by doing this.

They consist of creams or gels such as adapalene, tazarotene, and tretinoin. Topical retinoids have the potential to irritate skin and result in rashes. They can result in sunburns because using this product makes your skin more susceptible to UV rays.

If you use these lotions, you must wear sunscreen. Before choosing to take these medications, it is crucial to speak with your skin specialist.

Patients with acne only receive corticosteroid injections when their lesions have gotten so bad they could explode. As a result, the swelling lessens and the acne dries out quicker.

Isotretinoin is used to treat cystic acne and severe forms of acne. This is only for the treatment of complex acne issues and serious situations.

While successful in treating acne, oral contraceptives do have certain drawbacks. They are not intended for female smokers, ladies over the age of 35, or females who have blood coagulation issues.

Oral contraceptives reduce the extra glandular output, which in turn controls hormones to prevent acne.

TREATMENTS FOR ACNE AND HORMONE BALANCE

The development of acne is significantly influenced by hormones. Both the female and male hormones oestrogen and androgen play a role in the development of acne.

The release of these hormones coincides with puberty, menstruation, and pregnancy. This explains why a higher proportion of women than men have acne.

There are various ways to achieve a healthy hormone balance. These include maintaining a healthy weight, managing stress, drinking enough water, and exercising frequently.

The extra hormones and hazardous chemicals must be eliminated from your body. The kidneys and liver typically carry out this function.

You must realise, too, that these organs cannot perform their functions well if you eat poorly. You should have a balanced diet so that your body may get the nutrients it needs and function properly.

An ingredient that is present in excess will eventually cause the loss of another and damage your body's systems. Your skin will consequently be harmed by this.

The usage of antioxidants, which help to balance hormones and purify the blood of dangerous pollutants, is one of the natural remedies.

Additionally, attempting to consume a lot of water and avoiding caffeine might help prevent acne outbreaks. Exercise frequently, stay away from fried foods, and steer clear of stress and worry. All of these actions tend to limit the release of extra hormones and stop acne from developing.

To lessen imperfections, corticosteroids are useful. However, taking too many of these medications can also be detrimental, so you should always talk to your doctor before doing so.

Hormone equilibrium is best achieved through organic mechanisms. They promise excellent outcomes and pose no chance of negative side effects.

THE IDEAL ACNE NUTRITIONAL DIET

It is highly recommended for people with acne to eat a lot of fresh fruits and vegetables in their diet. To keep your system flushed out and toxin removal from your system ongoing, make it a point to drink a lot of water frequently. You only need eight to ten glasses per day.

Focusing on adding an antioxidant and fibre-rich diet is another smart move.

These are dietary components that will maintain your skin fit and healthy, allowing you to look and feel fantastic.

Protein is another element that is highly regarded for fighting acne. Health professionals believe that vitamin A is a powerful tool in the fight against acne.

Echinacea and Oregon grapes

These two herbs are particularly effective in boosting the immune system in your body and will also help reduce germs that are known to precipitate or worsen acne outbreaks.

HOW TO FIGHT AGAINST ACNE.

You need to build a system that includes a healthy diet and adhering to a routine that incorporates acne-fighting factors into your everyday life to regularly manage and remove acne.

Keep to this regimen until your acne is completely under control. It takes time and work to treat acne, but if you use the techniques in this manual, you will be well on your way to getting rid of acne for good.

You should feel and look your best. You can permanently control acne by doing your homework, talking to a skincare professional, and making small dietary and environmental changes.

SOME FOOD THAT PREVENTS ACNE

Foods that are good for the skin include:
yellow and orange fruits and vegetables such as carrots, apricots, and sweet potatoes
spinach and other dark green and leafy vegetables
turkey
blueberries
whole-wheat bread
brown rice
Nuts
Tomatoes
pumpkin seeds
 Peas, lentils and beans
salmon, mackerel, and other kinds of fatty fish
Quinoa

www.ingramcontent.com/pod-product-compliance
Lightning Source LLC
Chambersburg PA
CBHW051712250726
48653CB00007B/2986